Beat Cancer Before it Beats You!!!

Copyright 2013-Thomas T.

All rights reserved. This book is protected by the copyright laws of the United States of America. This book may not be copied, reprinted, stored in a retrieval system, or transmitted in any form or by any means, electronic, mechanical, recording or other for commercial gain or profit. The use of short quotations or occasional page copying for personal or group study is permitted and encouraged.

Copyright of images obtained from Google.

DEDICATION

This book is dedicated to my wife, Maria, and children Elizabeth, Antony, Charlie and Sheril, and to you, the reader, blessings indeed from God Almighty.

Acknowledgements

It started a few years ago with the leader of BWW, the late Mr. Bill Britt, stating that the state of our health can be ascertained by testing the saliva. Thank you Bill, I know you are enjoying the Eternal Bliss.

This book would not have been possible without the review and comments by Dr. Kalind Bakshi, Vascular Surgeon and Health Coach. Dr. Bakshi did his own pH test and convinced himself that more study is warranted. He also conducted research to find clinical studies related to urine pH and provided many comments to open up this book to the medical community.

Cover design by- Sheril James

Contents

Foreword

Introduction

1. The touch of a button-The story of my 22-year old nephew.
2. Who are we and what is our worth?
3. We all have cancer cells in our bodies
4. You are not allowed to swim in an acidic pool, but are your organs swimming in an acidic pool?
5. The story of a kidney cancer patient and a remarkable discovery
6. The story of an iced tea and my big lesson in health
7. The wisdom of our mothers and the gift of nature
8. You have just 30 days to live-Fighting the war with cancer
9. Is there a scientific basis for testing urine pH?
10. A call for research
11. A roadmap for your good health and happiness
12. Conclusion

Appendix A -Test results of pH variation and RBC in the urine of a kidney cancer patient-Feb 2012
Appendix B- pH tabulation form for base lining
Appendix C- Follow up test results in Jan. 2013 of the case study in Appendix A
Bibliography

The statements made in this book have not been evaluated by the Food and Drug Administration. The products mentioned in this book are not intended to diagnose, treat, cure or prevent any disease.

Foreword
Dr. Kalind Bakshi M.D. Vascular Surgeon and Health Coach

Many of us have heard the phrase take the "Acid Test". From the standpoint of Human Physiology, an acid environment indeed is a test.

Louis Pasteur was the Father of the Germ theory of disease who championed his thought processes to get deep seated roots into the minds of generations to come. The evidence? According to new federal reports in 2011, human antibiotic's use was over 7 million pounds in the U.S. and for livestock, over 29 million pounds! It is no wonder that the pharmaceutical world is consumed in a battle with resistant organisms, with billions of dollars!

Alexander Fleming , the discoverer of penicillin, in his Nobel prize speech in 1945 warned "misuse of penicillin will lead to the emergence of bacterial resistance".

It is therefore ironic that while a bacteria "responds" to a change in its environment, the very principle of Homeostasis- the "Milieu Interieur" espoused by Claude Bernard, a famous French Physiologist, gets overlooked by many. It is said that Pasteur acknowledged on his deathbed that Claude Bernard- his contemporary- was indeed right, that the internal environment is indeed important in disease process - not just the bacteria.

So how does all this tie into the Acid Test we are talking

about? We now know well that our blood pH is very tightly regulated between 7.38-7.42, barely allowing the maximum outside range of 7.35 to 7.45. All enzymatic processes start getting affected adversely particularly in an acidic environment. This indeed results in a "state of illness" and a not- so-pleasant environment for cells to grow, thrive or even survive. Chronic disease would be an expected outcome. Genetic mutation in response to the long standing environmental change, as we see in bacterial resistance, may also lead to cancer.

Thomas T. brings out this important aspect through a detailed case study with his dad, along with personal consistent and disciplined observation over the last 11 years. Thomas chose to study and follow what he calls the Litmus test of urine pH to determine our body's day today, nay- moment to moment- environment. Acidic pH is detrimental to the metabolic machinery. In a recent study from the University of Texas in 2007, low urine pH was closely associated with Metabolic Syndrome.
There have been eight chronic diseases linked with ongoing low pH. Currently, we have methods such as serum pH through arterial blood analysis available for accurate assessment. However, its usefulness is limited due to availability, invasiveness, expense and required expertise. Urine pH is simple, doable and predictable as Thomas has demonstrated to reflect a healthy lifestyle or lack of it. Unlike the 24- hour urine pH that was the format in the Texas study, this is a spot litmus test closely related to a lifestyle event, such as supplements, type of foods etc. Followed consistently, it has the potential of detecting early problems, maintaining a healthy "milieu"/ lifestyle and possibly even prevents chronic illnesses through its adjustment. Can it help alter a disease process? Can it help change its prognosis? What happens with someone who has

chronic kidney disease?   The most unanswered question - can it help "cure"?

This book is written for the everyday individual and it shows the author's passion to bring a useful tool to the community of self-help individuals. It is also a plea to the Medical community to continue further scientific evaluation with appropriate data collection.
On a personal note, I followed Thomas's protocol and also found a close correlation of my urine pH with my own intake/ lack thereof of supplements, type of foods etc.

This book is presenting a strong argument to study a larger number of people in different aspects of physiology as well as disease.
As a health coach, the area of most help that one can offer would be promoting a healthy lifestyle as well as establishing accountability & consistency with anyone interested in bringing about the positive shift of the milieu - both external as well as internal.

Introduction

We go through life only once and for a very short time. We gain valuable experience that, I feel, should be shared with others so that their lives can be affected in a positive way.

My goal in writing this book is to share with you something valuable that can help you personally and through you, many others. I will share personal stories that led me to an amazing discovery. The discovery led me to collaborative efforts with Dr. Kalind Bakshi to do research and find many clinical studies as shown in chapter 9. *My call for action is to the medical community to conduct further research.* While the research proceeds, you can help yourself by doing a simple test at home. I have been doing it for more than 11 years which helped with the discovery as shown in chapter 5. It taught me how to be proactive in the fight against cancer and other degenerative diseases.

In a clinical study of 24 hour urine pH, *"Low urine pH: A novel feature of the Metabolic Syndrome (1)"* **the authors** conclude that unduly acidic urine is a feature of metabolic syndrome. It is also found to be associated with the degree of insulin resistance. Metabolic syndrome is the name for a group of risk factors that raise your risk for heart disease and other health problems, such as diabetes and stroke. There are many more clinical studies referred to in chapter 9 for those who are interested in further research. The data that I show in appendix A and C is so convincing that we should seek more research for the betterment of humanity.

The paper *"Your Urine is Not a Window to Your Body (2),"* **questions the validity of urine pH measurements and the final conclusion was to take calcium and vitamin D along**

with daily dose of fruits and vegetables. The article was mainly against the claims that are apparently not substantiated, according to this article, in an effort by some to sell their products.

Please note that I am not trying to sell you any products through this book. I do take organic supplements which helped achieve the powerful results shown in the Appendix. Certain regulations even forbid me from giving the name of the company or its products

Cancer is one of the degenerative diseases, along with heart disease, diabetes, and there are many more. After over 11 plus years of readings, studies and pH testing, I came across an amazing discovery. That discovery alone made me want to write this book.

My Dad was diagnosed with kidney cancer at the age of 89. Because of his age surgery was ruled out. We were told to do nothing and have the cancer take its toll. I found that he was bleeding through the urine and was able to stop the bleeding by increasing his urine pH from 5.5 to 7. Acidic urine was hurting him internally.

The simple test that I suggest is to check your urine pH using litmus paper. This will give you a visual feedback about your health. Once you know where you are, you can take simple steps to safeguard your health.

Exposure to the Health and Wellness Industry is what helped me discover the urine pH test and how to manage acidity in your body. By manipulating acidity of the body, I was able to control the effect of my father's disease. That alone motivated me to write down my thoughts for the benefit of you, my reader. God forbid, if you or anyone else you know have succumbed to cancer, I will show you how you can fight it out as shown in chapter 8.

What is pH?

pH stands for potential hydrogen. The pH of water is 7 and is considered neutral. Anything below 7 is acidic and anything above 7 is alkali. The body is largely made up of water, a medium which is useful in allowing nutrients to be transported. Blood pH is very sensitive, staying within the narrow range of 7.38 to 7.42. In an alkaline state, the body has an abundance of oxygen. In an acidic state, our body has inadequate oxygen.

From a layman's perspective, to enjoy optimal health, it seems better to have more oxygen than less oxygen, doesn't it? Once you know the status of your body pH, I will suggest steps to maintain your body pH to be in a safe range by balancing the three pillars of optimal health.
The three pillars of Optimal Health are

1. *Lifestyle*
2. *Nutrition*
3. *Supplementation*

If you manage your pH on a regular basis by balancing the above pillars, you can reduce the risk for contracting diseases. There is no need for a prescription for the test and no co-pay is required. You will also learn to fight disease much better, in case you or anyone in your circle of influence have succumbed to it.

My journey towards this book started at the deathbed of my 22 year old nephew in December 2002. Ever since then I started to study more. When I heard at a conference that a simple test of our acidity could give an indication of our health, I decided to consider it seriously. Being an electrical engineer, I have learned a lot about input and output. You know that the output will be bad if the input is bad. It is just the law of nature. If we feed our body with acid forming foods, our urine pH will be acidic. This is just basic chemistry. If we feed our body with alkalizing foods, mostly fruits and vegetables, our urine pH will be alkaline.

The three pillars of Optimal Health will affect body pH on a dynamic basis. After many years of pH testing, I can say with 100% conviction that before we fall victim to degenerative diseases, it will show warning signs. Acidic urine is one of those signs and it can be tested in the privacy of your own home. The test is very simple, inexpensive, and is supported by scientific evidence as I will show later on in chapter 9.

"Take the litmus test "

I have always heard the term, "take the litmus test" in other contexts. Imagine taking the actual litmus test, on a regular basis, to maintain and protect your health! I have been carrying litmus paper ever since I left my nephew's death bed for self testing and for sharing it with others. I believe that the pH test is our way of monitoring the status of our health on a daily basis. It will prompt us to take corrective action by making adjustments in lifestyle, nutrition, and by taking supplementation, which I will elaborate later on.

Collecting the pH "evidence"

Getting the evidence to convince you is very easy when you set your mind to it. May I suggest a project for you to help in you seeking the evidence? Just fill out the pH form in appendix B for one day without changing anything. I am looking for readings when it is out of balance with acidic urine and another day when it is in balance with the pH being in the proper range. When you see the color change from acidic to neutral and will also be able to feel better, you will be convinced.

If you care to share your pH data with me, it will turn out to be a valuable set of information that will be of help to a lot of people. All you need to do is to fill out the pH tracking form with age, sex and notes about the medication and medical situation if any. You don't need to give your personal information. You may email the data to bodyphdata@gmail.com

What to do after reading this book

Just reading this book will not change your life in a positive way. But reading and starting to test your body pH will be a good beginning towards your optimal health. Once you are personally convinced that maintaining proper pH is critical for your health, you will be empowered to share the good news. It will help many people out there who may possibly fall victim to cancer and other degenerative diseases. The moment you start sharing this with others, you will start making a positive difference in their lives. That will lead you to help a multitude of others and make a tremendous positive impact in our society.

Beat Cancer Before it Beats You

Many live life thinking that some of their family and friends will develop cancer, suffer, and have an untimely death. My message is that there is something we can do to change that.

If your urine pH tests acidic, it is an indication that you are cutting short on at least one of the three pillars of Optimal Health.

1. You are not getting proper exercise.

2. Your eating habits trend towards acid forming foods. (See the food chart in chapter 6 to see where your favorable foods are on the pH scale.)

3. You are not taking the proper supplements to maintain proper body pH.

Over the years I have seen many people with acidic urine. Many were normal "healthy" adults. Many were cancer patients. Unfortunately some of them are no longer with us. I have not seen a single cancer patient without highly acidic urine. If you have highly acidic urine, it does not mean that you have a degenerative disease. I tested myself many times with high acidity, but I elected not to stay in that stage for too long.

You could see many testimonies online and you don't have to believe them. But I am sure, your test results will be so convincing that you will believe in it and take action. *All we are looking for is a state of good health, by following the three pillars of Optimal Health, and tying that with a litmus test, a visual feedback from your body.*

Beat Cancer Before it Beats You

There are no secrets.

There are no secrets to good health. Your mom has told you, I am sure, to eat your vegetables. You know that when you exercise your muscles regularly, they will perform much better. Your heart, the most important muscle in your body, is no exception. When you are exercising your heart muscles, it works more and makes it stronger. While doing so, your lungs work more and your entire body gets rejuvenated.

We often fall short in many ways with exercise and nutrition. That is where supplements fill the void big time. My study found that it is impossible for me to maintain a neutral urine pH without proper supplementation.

Do supplements help? Of course, they do. Organic vitamins are the best for our body, despite the increased cost. They provide the plant nutrients which are proven to reduce our risk to diseases. It reminds me of a comment I heard: "chemotherapy is very expensive."

Chapter 1

The touch of a button-The story of my 22 year old nephew.

I am staring at the screen monitoring the several vital signs of my nephew, who is gasping for breath. It was only a few months ago that I saw the energetic young man playing basketball with my son. We were celebrating his astounding recovery from a bone marrow transplant after fighting leukemia for almost 11 years.

As I stood beside his bed, I could hear the sound of his ventilator struggling along with the young man to help pump his lungs with enough oxygen to keep him alive. Every so often the beeps from the monitors would break the silence. The monitors have so much data which I did not understand. Now I know what some of those numbers mean. For example, the blood oxygen level is supposed to be close to 100. But for my nephew, it was never that high. I overheard his doctor talk about acidosis. Several times a day, the nurse took blood for analysis of about 44 items. The one time I checked, only 11 out of the 44 parameters were in the normal range.

A few hours before I arrived in the hospital, my nephew was at the verge of death. I was told that his blood oxygen level dropped to 70 compared to that of a healthy person's 98 or above. His medical staff worked frantically to bring him back to life. He had overcome death several times.

Is it Fate?

Ironically, leukemia could not get him for years, but two pints of blood from a transfusion instead of the regular one pint collapsed his lungs along with his and his family's worldly dreams.

Life or Death Decision

X-rays revealed air build up in his lungs, which needed to be taken out using a surgically inserted tube. The doctors in a meeting suggested that the chances of survival were 1 to 2% and indirectly discouraged the procedure. It was a decision of life and death. We all knew well that he had defeated such odds many times before.

It was a tense meeting with the doctors. On one side was the helpless mother whose request not to give him two pints of blood was ignored by the doctor in charge. On the other side was the angry dad who fumed at the doctors. I was able to get everyone to hold hands and pray to seek Eternal help in our fight to keep him alive. By the end of the meeting, it was decided to go on with the procedure. After all, how could we take away the chance for him to stay alive?

The Bedrock Principles

It was only a few weeks prior, while being hospitalized, that he had participated in an essay competition on Principle Centered Leadership. He wrote that Faith, Hope and Courage were his bedrock principles.

Throughout their hard times, the strength that the family had was their faith in Jesus. A few days earlier, he had received an interview call from Harvard. He was excited about going to college, especially Harvard, and told his family to get an extension for one week. He never gave up hope.

The touch of a button

It was early in the morning of Dec 2, 2002. We kept a vigil at his bedside. I had been staring at all the life support systems for 2 days. I often dozed off and the loud beeps kept me up. The medical staff did a tremendous job under a very difficult situation. But the monitor that showed his vital signs continued to report bad news. His heart that pumped for the last 22 years was beginning to give up. The lungs that oxygenated his blood had been damaged beyond recovery, depriving him of the oxygen that he needed. I stood there in awe watching the monitor, thanking God for the good health I am blessed with. His parents stood by his side with prayerful vigilance.

The nurse came over and touched a button. All of the sudden, all the lights on the monitors went off. The mere touch of a button entered the 22 year old into the presence of God, his maker. Though heart breaking for us humans, it must have been a time of celebration in Heaven to greet the hero. His worldly struggles were over and he had claimed his eternal reward. He had left a legacy in this world, a legacy of Faith, Hope and Courage, the words that he wrote just a few days before.

Chapter 2

Who are we and what is our worth?

Standing at the bedside of my nephew and watching what he was going through, I had to appreciate my good health and the workings of the amazing human body.

Our body can perish if we are deprived of oxygen for a few minutes. Can you imagine yourself struggling to breathe, being unable to get any oxygen? The human body is glorified in many ways because there is life in that body. You take life out of the body and it will rot in no time. Did we have any control over our entrance into this world? Do we have any way to control our exit from this world? The only thing we can control is what we do with our God given life during the time that we are alive. God has given us complete control over the choices that we make.

Scientists estimate that our brain can perform calculations equivalent to several million of the most powerful computers currently available. Our brain controls all our actions, both good and bad, affecting everything that we do.

If we had an expensive sports car, I am sure we would use super gasoline, not regular gasoline. If we care so much about a car, can you put a dollar value to our body?

Often we lead unhealthy lifestyles, as we don't exercise properly nor watch what we eat. As a result, our body tends to become acidic. In layman's terms, our body does not have enough oxygen, the ideal energy needed to sustain optimal health. We live on with an acidic body and we don't even know it. We rely on doctors whom we visit as a last resort and sometimes too late. They give us results that are not easily comprehended and we end up taking a handful of prescription medications, with side effects that we do not even know.

I will show you a simple test, the test of the pH of your urine, revealing to you about the three pillars of Optimal Health-Lifestyle, Nutrition and Supplementation. Now is the time to be proactive and find out if you are at balance. Once you make the changes, the results are easily measurable. It all shows up in the color of the litmus paper. Our goal is to make the litmus paper look dark green, not yellow or light green, when you test your urine. Isn't that amazingly simple? Please don't let the simplicity confuse you. Start testing and you will know soon how simple it is and how you can take complete control of your health.

I was told by a reputable nutritionist that everyone has cancer cells in their body. The next chapter will cover that story.

Chapter 3

"We all have cancer cells in our bodies."

I am at the office of a New York State Board certified Dietitian/Nutritionist along with my sister who was diagnosed with breast cancer.

I am a firm believer in nutrition but did not want to test my theory on my younger sister. I wanted to rely on his over 50 years of experience working with supplementation to fight the harrowing disease, in tandem with the treatment recommended by the medical industry. In fact, this was the only time that I met with someone who knows about nutrition and who works with medical doctors in their typical routine of chemotherapy, radiation etc.

During the interview he said something that I will never forget. "We all have cancer cells in our body. In your sister's case, there are millions of cancer cells, but we may only have a few hundred. The big difference is that our immune system keeps it in check but in your sister's case, her immune system has failed to protect her". I do not have scientific evidence to support the above. But the statements make perfect sense to me.

That day I walked out of the office with a set of products and a pH test kit, with a goal to build up her immune system from that day on. "Time was of the essence", like what people say. If we know what to do, why would we delay it, especially when it is about dealing with a disease like cancer? It cost me more than $500 that day but I did not care. When it comes to cancer, it is a life and death situation. I wanted to provide the best for my sister. As usual, I checked her urine pH and found it to be highly acidic. But I was delighted to see it change from acidic to neutral with calcium and vitamin D3 supplementation.

She went through the normal routine of chemotherapy. What we did differently was providing the many supplements to boost her immune system. The nutritionist suggested that all supplementation be stopped 2 days before chemotherapy. Immediately after chemotherapy our body will start rebuilding process, which is exactly when we need to provide the best nutrients. Our body, the amazing gift from God, will rebuild itself under ideal conditions. Doctors suggest that you take foods that are rich in protein during chemo. Unfortunately, sick patients cannot eat properly due to side effects.

How many people have you seen go through the terrible side effects of chemo? You can find some tips in chapter 9 about how to fight the war with cancer using the power of nature.

Imagine being able to help reduce the side effects.

Imagine being able to boost the health.

It is ironic that we balance the pH of swimming pool water on a daily basis but we don't even think about our body pH balance. Read the next chapter about a related story.

Chapter 4

You are not allowed to swim in an acidic pool, but are your organs swimming in an acidic pool?

We have a pool at home and we have enjoyed many days of family fun. The most memorable was the night before when our marine son was deployed to Iraq for his first of three tours of duty. I had just opened the pool and even borrowed water from our neighbor to fill it in a hurry. But before the bunch of teens jumped in, I had to check the pH of the water. If the water was acidic, I will not allow them to swim in it. So I had to rush to the pool supply store to get pH Plus. Reading the ingredients, I found that they are granules of calcium. It reminded me of my chemistry class. Whenever a mineral is added to an acid solution, a chemical reaction takes place. The acid is neutralized and the pH of the water increases. Depending on the amount of calcium that was added, it could go above 7. A PH of 7.2 to 7.8 is considered ideal for a pool for us to swim in.

I am concerned about the acidity of the water that my children swim in. Do we know that many of us feast on acidic food, don't exercise enough and live our life with an acidic body? Acidosis hurts us gradually and leads us to all sorts of degenerative diseases and we don't even know it.

Beat Cancer Before it Beats You

We take care of our swimming pool more earnestly than our own body. Do you know the pH of the fluids that our organs are swimming in?

Take this simple test. Go to a party and eat all that your heart desires. Have your soda and alcohol too, if you would like. The next day, check the pH of your urine in the privacy of your house. My guess is that your urine will test to be acidic, say around 5-6 on the pH scale. All you need is a roll of pH paper that is made for testing urine pH. You can order it from the web. Your pharmacy may also have them.

A few years ago my office had a health fair and there was one company giving away pH paper to the employees. I bought mine from Willner chemists for $15 about 10 years ago. For a family, it should last a year. That $15 was the best investment I have made in my family's health. Ever since my discovery of the way to manage body pH, I have tried to maintain it at a neutral state using calcium and vitamin D3. Believe it or not, I have found that it is not easy for me without supplements as I show below.

My pH Experiments

While writing this book, I ran out of pH paper for a few weeks. So I bought a new stock from Micro Essential Lab.

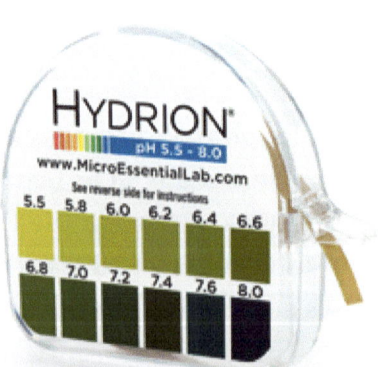

I run out of them very fast as I share the good news and the pH paper with everyone who is willing to listen. So I decided to do a baseline once again. That night we had rice, fried fish and some special relishes for dinner but no fruits and vegetables. I took regular vitamins but not Vitamin D3. The next morning I am ready to start my baseline. I intentionally did not take any vitamins in the morning. I found myself at pH 6, in an acidotic state. During the day I repeated the test every two hours. My pH even went down to 5.5 immediately after a meal bar with 15 grams of sugar in it. I had no vitamins in my office and so I bought Red Zinger tea, my favorite while in the office. My pH jumped from 5.5 to 6.2 in an hour. At home, during dinner, I took vitamin D3 and calcium in addition to my regular organic vitamins, balanced health and fruits and vegetables tablet. The next morning, my pH was at 6.2 again. I took Vitamin D3, and Calcium and a few others, the usual morning routine. I was delighted to see my pH jump to 7.2 and again during lunch, to 7.4.

Some of the readings state that the urine pH is always acidic in the morning, which I have confirmed myself. Recently I experimented with some vegetable juice and found that the best way to alkalize in the morning is to drink vegetable juice at night. You will wake up with a pH close to neutral, unlike the effect of traditional food.

Imagine getting the news that your dad has cancer and because of his age the medical community suggested to do nothing. My little education in pH testing helped me big time. The next chapter is the story that led to a remarkable discovery.

Chapter 5

The story of a Kidney cancer patient and a remarkable discovery.

My Dad, aged 90, enjoyed very good health for 73 years, living in India. He stayed very active, walking every day for about an hour, a routine developed to go to work. At age 73 he immigrated to the United States and there ended his "active" life and good eating habits. At age 76, he developed clogging of the arteries and had a stent put in. Afterwards I put him on protein powder, omega 3 supplements with 1500 mg of EPA, calcium and magnesium with vitamin D and multi vitamin-multi mineral supplements. Occasionally I checked his urine pH and maintained it at neutral. About three years ago he moved back to India. In January 2012, he was diagnosed with kidney cancer during a routine medical checkup. Because of his age, doctors did not recommend surgery. We were told to just wait and see. "Doctor, is there anything that we can do nutritionally?" was my question. He said that there was nothing that could be done.

Having experimented with body pH for many years, I decided to do my own testing. I found that my dad's urine was highly acidic at pH 5.5, the lowest I can measure with my litmus paper. My online research told me that the symptoms of kidney cancer are blood in urine, weight loss and fever. So the next thing I could do in India as a layman was to do a lab test of the urine. The test showed that there were traces of blood in his urine.

I knew that taking vitamin D3 and calcium had changed my urine pH from acidic to neutral many times over the years. So, I gave him Vitamin D3 in addition to the Calcium that he was taking occasionally. The next time I checked, the urine pH was neutral at 7. I took another sample of the urine for analysis in a lab. *Amazingly the traces of blood disappeared.* I was so thrilled to find out that by managing the pH of the urine, I could stop the loss of blood through the urine, a symptom of kidney cancer. I thanked God almighty for the blessing.

I got so excited and wanted to find out more. So I continued the pH test by giving him different liquids and other supplements. You could see the charts that I made with my notes in the Appendix A. Through many pH tests and lab tests I found that his condition would require double the dose of D3 than what is recommended for a normal adult. That was the pattern we were following as I wrote this chapter in Nov 2012.

Status of health after a year of detection of kidney cancer.

A year after my discovery, I went back to India with my entire family to celebrate the engagement of our daughter Elizabeth. I was blessed to find my dad physically active as usual. We had a wonderful celebration and counted all our blessings. He had been on Calcium & Magnesium and Vitamin D3 for the last year. But it was questionable as to how punctual he was in taking the supplements. So I did 5 different urine analyses on five consecutive samples along with the pH readings. I was shocked to find traces of blood in all the samples. The best pH reading that I got was a 6.2. I was very much concerned and personally took charge of the supplements and made sure that he took the same dosage, 4000 IU of vitamin D3 and calcium supplements that I suggested the year before. Early in the morning and also around 8am, I took two samples and was delighted to find that his urine pH had returned to 7. So I rushed the samples to the lab and gladly found no traces of blood in both samples, proving again that by proper supplementation of D3 and Calcium, his urine pH can be made neutral. That process stopped the loss of blood through his urine, a symptom of his kidney cancer. By manipulating the pH balance of his body I was able to control the effects of his medical condition, the dreaded kidney cancer, once again, a year after he was diagnosed.

This is where I stop as I am only an engineer and make my plea to the medical community.

1. Please start charting the pH of cancer patients as well as those who have other medical conditions and compare them with those of healthy adults.

2. Collect data to study the correlation between pH of urine and different medical situations. It may lead to enhanced treatments. A body that is pH balanced may be more conducive to different treatments as some clinical studies (1) (2) suggest.

We go through life and learn major lessons along the way. The next chapter will cover one of my big lessons in health.

Chapter 6

The Story of an Iced Tea and my big lesson in health

Imagine a health professional, giving a talk on Total Health, reading the ingredients on an iced tea. His facial expression changes, he takes the bottle and throws it into the garbage can without even opening it. I was baffled, wondering why he threw away the iced tea that he paid for. My kids love it and I was used to buying it all the time. He explained that the "offensive" ingredient was high fructose corn syrup. That seminar was a wakeup call for me and prompted me to study the processed food industry and its effects on the body's pH balance. Many drinks have a high level of acidity and come with a lot of calories. In layman's terms they rob the body of oxygen and compromise our health. How can we know? The answer is very simple: *Just check the pH of your urine.*

My big lesson in health

Attending the health seminar, I proudly stated that I am in good health, because I take the organic vitamins. The instructor retorted. "Tom, just taking vitamins won't cut it. There are three things to focus on for maintaining optimal health." He went on to elaborate the three things. Ever since that time I have been talking to people about it and has discovered a simple and inexpensive test that anyone can do themselves to authenticate whether the three are in balance. They are the three pillars for Optimal Health that I wrote earlier. To reinforce, let me focus more on them.

1. Lifestyle
2. Nutrition
3. Supplementation

Let us review it one by one in detail.

1. *Lifestyle.*

There are many questions that we need to ask ourselves about us and our health.

- Am I aware as to how unique I am? There is no one like us in the whole world and no one ever will exist. We have a unique purpose in life. Have I discovered it? If not, are we seeking it?
- Am I taking good care of my amazing body, the gift from God?
- Am I exercising at least 30 minutes every day to keep my body in good shape?
- Am I in control of stress or, is stress in control of me?
- Am I in good relationship with God?
- Am I in good relationship with my family?
- Am I in good relationship with my friends and colleagues?
- Am I living my life with a positive attitude?

There is only one life to live. We need to live in harmony with everyone around us. That will lead us to a healthy, happy and peaceful life.

2. *Nutrition*

You are what you eat. How are your eating habits? As the chart below shows, every food has a pH value associated with it. If you consume acidic foods, your urine pH will be acidic. If you eat more of the alkalizing food, your urine pH will be 7 or more indicating that your body has more oxygen. If you review the list carefully, the fruits and vegetables fall in the alkalizing category. Our taste buds seem to prefer acid forming foods. White sugar, white bread, white pasta and white rice are just not the healthy choices. It is alright to eat them as long as it is in moderation and we manage to keep the urine pH neutral.

Like your mom always said, eat your vegetables. Take a look where hamburgers are on the chart below. Are you surprised? Do you think the little lettuce on your hamburger will do the job of giving you adequate vegetables? I don't think there is a chance. Why not start your experiment with the different foods, especially all the different colors, and at the same time chart your urine pH. You will be convinced of the connection between urine pH and the food chart below. This is where your discovery will really start.

A review of our Food habits

Foods are classified in to two different types, acid-forming and alkali-forming. As you see in the chart below, most high protein foods such as meat, fish, poultry and carbohydrates are acid-forming whereas fruits and vegetables are alkali-forming in the body.

Acid-Forming foods	**Meats & Fish**	pork, veal, hamburgers
		polished rice, beef, oysters, crab, lobster
		shrimp, ham, turkey, chicken, coffee & tea
		fresh water fish, eggs, liquor, chocolate
	Grains	hard cheese, ocean fish, natural and wild rice
		beer, wine, pasta, spaghetti
		whole grain breads, margarine, nuts, butter, cream
	Dairy	soft cheese, whey
		cow's milk, goats milk

Beat Cancer Before it Beats You

Alkali-Forming foods	Fruits & Vegetables	potatoes, lentils, onions, garlic, apples
		pears, bananas, oranges, raisins
		beans, olives, molasses
		cabbage & lettuce
		greens, soy nuts, beets, celery, carrots
		tomatoes, dried figs
		lecithin, ginger, spinach
		cucumbers, radishes, squash

Source:- Google search.

3. Supplementation

Items 1 and 2 covered lifestyle and nutrition. When we fall short, we need supplementation to maintain pH balance and optimal health. When it comes to supplements, there are organic and inorganic choices. Organic vitamins come from plants and animals, whereas inorganic minerals come from soil and water.

I opt for supplements made from certified organic products. I take supplements to fill the void as there are many voids in our diet. The organic supplements provide the plant concentrates that we don't normally get from the synthetic vitamins. It is through the health and wellness industry that I learned about pH balance many years ago. During a training session I heard that the pH of your saliva can give you information about health. The idea intrigued me and I started the search by testing the pH of saliva and urine that resulted in the writing of this book.

How are you doing with the three pillars of optimal health?

The answer is very simple. The end result of your lifestyle, nutrition and supplementation habits show up in your urine pH. May I suggest the following? Before you even make any change to anything, please chart your body pH baseline. Start charting in the morning by testing and recording your urine pH every time you void for a day. Use the table in Appendix B to document. Don't worry, you have to do the baseline only once in your life. That will prove to be a good investment in your health. Once you know your baseline, compare it with the ideal values in the table.

Beat Cancer Before it Beats You

What I have seen over the years is that most likely you are in unsafe range as I was. That is exactly how my pool is if I don't treat it on a daily basis. In the case of the pool, all I do is to throw some calcium granules in on a regular basis. Our body requires a little more attention. When I find my pH to be acidic, the simple thing that I do is to take calcium and magnesium with vitamin D3. As you may know we are to get our vitamin D from sunlight. Unfortunately we don't spend enough time in the sun. So after a routine blood test, my doctor suggested that I take additional vitamin D3 because the calcium supplement that I take has only 100 IU of vitamin D. So I take 2000 IU of vitamin D3, a phenomenal product that can provide amazing protection.

If your urine pH tests to be acidic, there is nothing to worry. All you need is to take 2000 IU of D3 and calcium and test after 2 hours. You will be delighted to find that your urine pH has become neutral. *When the pH is neutral, I have found that I don't get acid reflux.* You may want to try it out too. I am sure you know many people who live with acid reflux. My hope is that you will be able to help them after learning about and doing the pH test.

From the knowledge of our body chemistry, blood in the pH range of 7.38 to 7.42, provide the abundance of oxygen to sustain life. There is more oxygen in the body when the body is in alkaline state than in acidic state. I can concur with what science says. If you eat more fruits and vegetables your body pH will become more alkaline. *Our moms may not have known the scientific explanation but they were right in stressing the importance of eating fruits and vegetables.*

Much has been written about degenerative diseases and how they start with acidity in the body. In simple words, diseases start from inadequate amounts of oxygen. This should bring up the idea of evidence based medicine. Of course I cannot make unsubstantiated claims. But I want to present to you my evidence, based on chemistry. My studies so far and actual pH readings provided results as shown in Appendix A and C which I feel should be studied further.

I am looking for medical doctors who can initiate more clinical studies. I had a pathologist who told me that they don't monitor the urine pH of cancer patients except prior to administering certain treatments. He admitted that it is a very simple thing to do. I hope and pray that many doctors all over the world will start to take urine pH tests of all the patients. Imagine if all those who read this were to do a baseline of urine pH in their current state. If they are not in the safe range based on pure chemistry, let them try to improve it and report the values with notes detailing how they managed to change their pH. That will provide sufficient amount of data for research.

Just by the nature of their profession, doctors are taught to treat diseases, after we get sick. In many cases it is too late and the price we pay is very high. *pH testing is all about preventing diseases before we fall victim to it*. In one test we will know about our lifestyle, food habits and supplementation. I was surprised to see all the clinical studies connecting urine pH and diseases including cancer as outlined in chapter 9.

I lovingly remember my nephew, a young and energetic man with a lot of passion for life. I was at his bedside when he took his last breath. Since then I have read a lot about what to do to possibly reduce the risk of cancer. There are many risk factors which are in our control. *In my opinion, it is possible to reduce your risk to cancer even if your risk is genetic. Nutrigenomics and Epigenetics are things that you would want to read to stay abreast of advancements.* Nutrients can play a major role in the gene expression.

We are all familiar with the age old saying "prevention is better than cure." I am sure you agree that you will do everything possible to avoid getting cancer.

I had a young doctor ask me a while ago. "What good is the pH test? Of course, if we eat pasta, rice etc your urine will test acidic". By his comment he was admitting that along with the pasta he is not going to have his fruits and vegetables. Many times, I have found myself feasting on an unbalanced meal. Now that I know about pH and supplements, I do take supplements to keep the balance right. *My objective in writing this book is to lead you to do the same by educating yourself so that you stay Healthy and help many others in your circle of influence stay healthy as well. Remember, we only have one life to live. If we don't share what we know within our circle of influence, some of them will never get the message.*

Chapter 7

The Wisdom of our Mothers and the Gift of Nature.

"Eat your vegetables" is something that my mom would say often. But I disliked most of the vegetables. Now that I have four of my own children I do understand my mom very well. Life experience taught all our moms to insist on children eating their vegetables. The food pyramid published by the FDA, Food and Drug Administration of the U.S. Government, stresses the importance of including fruits and vegetables in our diet.

Why do we need fruits and vegetables?

PHYTONUTRIENTS- the nutrients found in plants when consumed adequately can reduce risk of diseases. Let us look at the images of a few fruits and vegetables and compare them to the images of our organs.

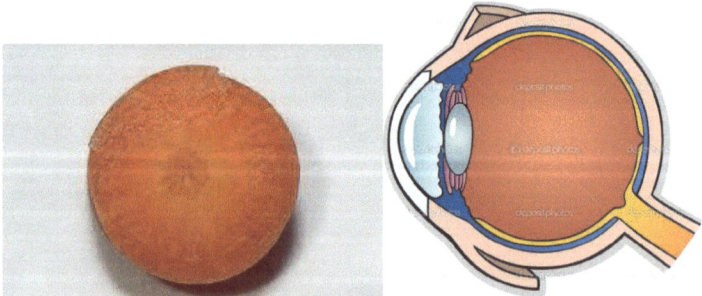

Compare the images of a human eye and a carrot. Everyone knows that carrots are good for the eyes.

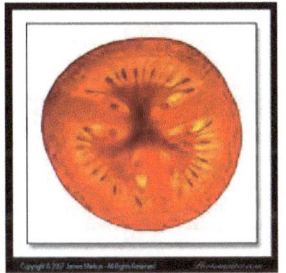 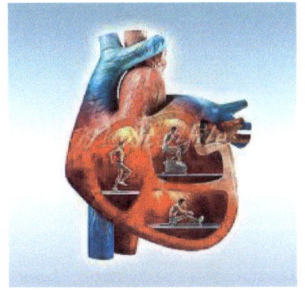

Now, let us compare the images of a human heart and a tomato. Is it any wonder that tomatoes are good for your heart?

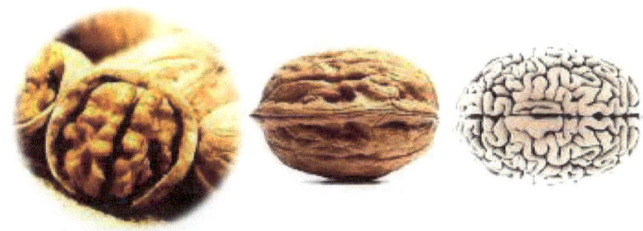

Courtesy- Google Images

What about a comparison of our brain and a walnut?

You can look at all the fruits and vegetables and compare them to our human body. God has intended them all for our healthy existence. He also gave us the power to choose.

If we don't learn from nature, we can learn from the food pyramid which says we should include 9 to 12 servings of fruits and vegetables every single day? When you do, you can have a healthy life. You can find many studies that point towards a reduction in the risk of cancer if our diet is rich in fruits and vegetables.

Even from a religious standpoint, Ezekiel 47:12 mentions the importance of fruits and vegetables, "their fruit will be for food, and their leaves for healing."

What do we do to get the fruits and vegetables?

Many people don't get adequate fruits and vegetables. In this hectic life, who has the time? So we try but often fail. I commend you if you get all that you need from fruits and vegetables, which will be the ideal. Did you know that we are supposed to eat fruits and vegetables of all colors? You can take an online color test and see how close you are to the ideal.

You may wonder as to how all this is going to help someone who has cancer. Please read on to find your answer in the next chapter.

Chapter 8

You have just 30 days to live- Fighting the war with cancer

"My doctor told me 28 years ago, you have just 30 days to live". I heard that from the instructor of the Iced Tea story during a health class. I have heard of many cases where doctors gave the remaining duration for someone's life. Unfortunately many patients take it as "God's word" and program their end of life as the doctor projected. In this case, my instructor did not give any credit to what his doctor said. 28 years later, he was teaching about the three pillars of optimal health that could safeguard anyone's health. Let me repeat them here again so that it gets into your memory.

- o **Lifestyle**
- o **Nutrition**
- o **Supplementation**

Fighting the war with cancer

Imagine going through cancer. It is a war, a life and death war, sometimes a "lonely" war. This is where the individual needs emotional support from people all around them while they fight the gruesome disease.

Beat Cancer Before it Beats You

Secrets to winning the war

Faith

The first and foremost is faith- faith in God almighty, faith in yourself, faith in the medical staff and faith in all the loved ones around you. When we believe that our body is the temple of God, a wonderful machine powered by the maker, the situation is only temporary. I believe that God has a purpose for my life in this world. We must identify that purpose and finish our task. So, have the Faith that we will finish our work that God has entrusted us in this wonderful world. The temporary situation could be a wake- up call.

But the secret to success in the war is to tap into the infinite resources of that ultimate power, Faith in God Almighty.

Hope

The second secret is hope, hope to accomplish things that we are destined to do. A human being with hope can make wonders happen, no matter what the circumstances are, especially when they tap into the ultimate power of God Almighty.

Courage

The third secret that my nephew wrote about was courage. We obtain courage automatically when we are blessed with Faith and Hope. The journey that we take in this world is not easy. Sometimes it becomes so difficult that many give up. But when the journey gets tough, having the faith that there is an infinite power as your resource, will rekindle your hope, and you will get the courage to move on with life, fighting it out, one day at a time, sometimes one moment at a time.

The Power of Spoken Word

Our sub conscious mind has amazing power that we can tap into using the power of our spoken words. Keep saying to yourself loudly many times a day "Every day in every way I am getting better and better." As a Christian I add to it "I can overcome all things through Christ who strengthens me". Whatever your religion is, say exactly what you want and it will happen. It is my belief that by speaking positively, we can tap into the power of the "Infinite Intelligence", God Almighty.

The mechanics of fighting the war with cancer

Once the mind is focused on the war, next will be the daily action steps. Here is a step by step plan, which I am hopeful will lead you to victory, which of course should be done in close consultation with your physician.

Step 1
Obtain a pH test kit, either from your pharmacy or online. I have used the one made by Micro Essential Laboratories for many years and found it to give consistent results. Please note that I do not have any business connection with them.

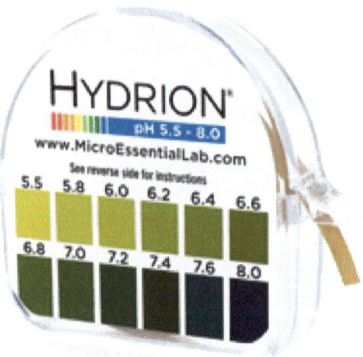

One close friend of mine flagged me about the accuracy of pH measurements between dipsticks and a pH meter (9). He cited a Mayo Clinic paper, dealing with accuracy while administering the Methotrexate treatment for cancer. The paper suggested not to alternate between dipstick and pH meter. Under the current circumstances, I suggest to keep it simple and economic by using a roll of litmus paper.
Note: High quality pH meters are very expensive and will require continuous calibration with a buffered solution and in my opinion this is not practical for average people. I can see its use in a clinical study.

Step 2

Base Lining of pH.
Start testing the urine pH every time you go, for one day and fill up the form in appendix B. Don't change anything that you are doing now. The goal is to find out exactly where you are without making any changes.

Step 3

Analyze the results.
Based on my reading and the test results of many, I am convinced that the ideal range you want to be is between 6.5 and 7.5. My dad was bleeding through the urine when his pH was below 6.5. One urologist told me that when they do the urine pH test, they do not worry about the low values, unless there is something medically wrong with the person. Further studies may prove otherwise.

Step 4

Balancing the body pH
If you are tested to be acidic, take 2000 IU of D3 and 200 mg of calcium and magnesium and test again. You will see the change with the pH moving up. Your goal is to take enough supplements to raise the pH to a range of 6.5 to 7.5. For those who worry about taking too much calcium, the litmus paper will warn you as it increase above 7.5.
So by continuous testing you will identify the dosage that you need to keep within the acceptable range of 6.5 to 7.5.

Step 5

Long term maintenance
You may ask "How long do I have to test myself?" You do it until you are confident that the test results are staying within the acceptable range.

What to do during Chemotherapy?

During chemotherapy, cancer cells are destroyed and along with this some healthy cells are also destroyed. The expectation is that the body will produce healthy cells. Protein is the basic building block of each and every cell in our body. Patients are asked to eat protein rich foods after chemo.

PDCAAS is a score of how absorption of protein is measured. It stands for Protein Digestibility Corrected Amino Acid score. A PDCAAS score of 1 is considered ideal. As the patient takes a good source of protein, their chance of recovery should be better, with fewer side effects.
I have many personal experiences of cancer patients getting better, much faster after taking the protein powder. In one case I was told that the patient did not need the blood transfusion after taking protein powder. Clinical studies of 24 hour urine pH along with the consumption of a good source of protein, calcium and vitamin D3 may provide valuable data.

I am hoping that enough people will start to volunteer for testing the pH when they go through chemo so that we can build enough data to support proper pH balancing even during chemo.

We need facts. I suggest that we take charge of our health and start testing the urine pH. What is ideal will be to get the baseline first. Once you know the baseline, do whatever you need to, to bring the urine pH between 6.5 and 7.5 and assess the health situation. Clinical studies hopefully will validate these numbers or modify them for effective treatment.

Beat Cancer Before it Beats You

Knowing what we know, I suggest that we select food from the alkalizing group. I will also take antioxidant complex, selenium complex and protein powder to re-build the cells and enough calcium and vitamin D3 to maintain the urine pH between 6.5 and 7.5. It is very important that we don't take too much calcium either. If we do, we will go into alkalosis. The best way is to make sure that the litmus paper does not turn dark blue.

Of course we have to do all these under the guidance of our physicians. Just in case the physician says NO, then it is your turn to ask some specific questions.

- How can I manage to get the urine pH between 6.5 and 7.5?
- Is there any harm in taking at least calcium and Vitamin D3?
- Is there any harm in taking the Protein Powder?

If they say that any of the things are harmful to the body, you may want to get a second opinion and then listen to the experts.

I have read in many places that cancer cells thrive in an acidic body. Without even knowing the mechanism behind it, I find it easy to agree because I know what acidity means from chemistry. It is the lack of oxygen. If lack of oxygen can kill you, abundance of oxygen should only help you. So do whatever you can to manage your body pH. Read chapter 5 about my dad's case of kidney cancer and how a dosage of 4000 IU of vitamin D3 stopped the traces of blood in his urine.

Beat Cancer Before it Beats You

The best research you can do is by yourself about your body pH. Once you discover the answer, work with your medical doctor to validate what you do.

When you regain your health, you will be so excited about it that you would want to share it with everyone around your circle of influence by teaching the three pillars of optimal health.

- **Lifestyle**
- **Nutrition**
- **Supplementation**

As per the pocket guide to Micronutrients in Health and Disease (10)there are dietary substances that act as promoters of cancer and other dietary substances that act as inhibitors of cancer.

Foods to be avoided by cancer patients.

Avoid high intake of fat, especially saturated fat from meat products, processed meats, burned or darkly browned foods, rancid fats, such as fat used repeatedly for deep fat frying, food preservatives, artificial food dyes, alcohol and heavily chlorinated drinking water. While fruits and vegetables are considered good for you, avoid the non-organic type. While fish is considered good, please do the research about the presence of toxic chemicals like mercury.

Foods that are to help cancer patients.

The foods that help cancer patients are fiber rich foods, whole grains, bran, fruits, legumes, seeds, dark green and yellow-orange vegetables, broccoli, Brussels sprouts, cabbage, cauliflower, fresh beets, carrots, asparagus, onions, garlic, calcium-rich foods, fresh fruit and fruit juices.

How can we find out the net result of our diet? Believe it or not, it shows up in the pH of your urine. So your best bet is the continuous pH testing of your urine until you know what the effect is while consuming different foods.

Vitamins to take after you have recovered.

Certified organic is one word that I would stress. The plant concentrates are provided in nature by our maker for our protection. Try to get the Best of Nature and the Best of Science.

In addition to calcium and vitamin D3, take Selenium, vitamin A, C and E, all anti oxidants, folic acid and vitamin B12.

I would get a roll of litmus paper and start testing the urine pH? It is one test that can give you good news and bad news. A dark green pH paper, (pH=7) will give you confidence and a sense of satisfaction that you are taking care of yourself well. The bad news could be that the pH paper is yellow or light yellow in color (pH=5 to6.2). The bad news is not that bad either as you can change it in about 2 hours by taking vitamin D3 and Calcium.

But if you don't test it, you will never know whether you are acidic or not. Of course your body will give you many symptoms of ill health. But we want to be proactive and hopefully prevent cancer or any other degenerative diseases or its reoccurrence.

Beat Cancer Before it Beats You

You may wonder as to what scientific evidence is available to help understand and commit to making the changes to improve our health. When I started the book, with the intention of sharing the test results, I was not aware of the many clinical data that is currently available. The next chapter will cover some of the scientific data that correlate urine pH and medical situations.

Chapter 9

Is there a scientific basis for testing urine pH?

My discovery of vitamin D3 and calcium, being able to stop the blood loss through urine of a kidney cancer patient was unexpected. With the help of Dr. Kalind and also through the internet, I was able to get more scientific data connecting urine pH and diseases. Let me present some of them to you.

1. The clinical journal of the American society of Nephrology (1) demonstrated a relationship between Metabolic Syndrome (MS) and low urine pH. Metabolic syndrome is the name for a group of risk factors that raises your risk for heart disease and other health problems, such as diabetes and stroke. What is noteworthy in the study is the increasing number of MS features with a decline in 24 hour urine pH.

2. The Journal of clinical Endocrinology and Metabolism (2) reported a study which concluded that patients with low–risk prostate cancer under active surveillance may benefit from vitamin D3 supplementation at 4000IU. This is the same exact dose that I used with my dad by testing the urine pH continuously, and stopping his bleeding through urine.

3. A conference paper (3) presented at the second International Acid-Base Symposium, Nutrition-Health-Disease in Munich, Germany, September 2006, dealt with

the issue of the populations in the US and UK not getting the health benefits of well recognized fruits and vegetables, a proven way to prevent cancer. The paper identified dipstick measurement of urine pH as a potential Biomarker, which reflects the acid-base load of the diet. As per the study, the dipstick measures of urine pH are simple and rapid and could provide a feedback mechanism during dietary change.

4. A service of the U.S. National Institutes of Health provides information on many clinical trials during the many stages of a trial. One completed trial (4) reports that vitamin D and calcium supplementation can assume an important role in the treatment of type 2 Diabetes and in the <u>prevention of the disease in the 41 million Americans who are at risk of developing type 2 Diabetes</u>. I will show you in appendix A as to how vitamin D and calcium increased my dad's urine pH significantly.

5. The University of Pittsburg school of Medicine (5) reports that monitoring urinary pH during mytomycin C adjuvant treatment and modifying pH for urine alkalization may improve the therapeutic efficacy of mitomycin C instillation. Mitomycin is an anti-tumor antibiotic used specifically <u>in the treatment of cancer. It interferes with the multiplication of cancer cells.</u>

6. <u>Oxford Journal's</u> report on Carcinogenesis (6) suggests that urine pH, which is determined primarily by diet and body surface area, may be an important modifier of smoking and risk of bladder cancer. The study found that consistently acidic urine pH <=6 was associated with an increased risk of bladder cancer.

7. American Association for Cancer Research (7) refers to MTX therapy, a chemotherapy, which requires a highly alkaline urine pH of 7 or more. The study focused on the effect of urine pH on various beverages and found that yogurt, buttermilk and soda made the urine more acidic compared to tube feeding and orange juice which help alkalize the urine. Their goal was to identify foods to avoid and also identify foods that could raise the pH when taken in substantial amounts. This helped to make the therapy on an outpatient basis. The study ended up recommending against consuming yogurt, soda and buttermilk prior to chemotherapy.

8. As usual there is dissenting opinion. When I read the paper "Your Urine is Not a Window to Your Body (8) questioning the validity of the urine pH measurements, their final conclusion was to take calcium and vitamin D along with a daily dose of fruits and vegetables. This is the same conclusion of many studies. The article was mainly against the "claims" that are not "substantiated" in an effort by some to sell their products.

The evidence presented above leads to a potential for many more studies. The next chapter is an appeal to the medical community to embrace more studies with the expectation of enhancing the healthcare as well as taking proactive steps to prevent diseases.

Chapter 10

A call for research

Following are some questions that came to my mind after reading the clinical studies.

1. "Metabolic syndrome study" suggests that the higher the 24 hour urine pH, the lesser the metabolic symptoms. The highest 24 hour pH was 6.1. What could the effect be, if it was manipulated to be between 6.5 and 7.5? It could easily be achieved with the administration of D3 and calcium?

2. If 4000 IU of vitamin D3 is proven to be helpful for cancer patient, why not track the 24 hour urine pH of that group and compare that to healthy adults?

3 If chemotherapy mandates a urine pH of 7, can we study treatments of all other diseases and their effect by mandating the PH to be at 7?

4 If soda and buttermilk are found to reduce urine pH, and not recommended prior to chemotherapy, wouldn't it be a food to be totally avoided by cancer patients?

6 Why is it that all cancer patients that I tested have highly acidic urine?

7. The clinical studies in chapter 9 suggests
a correlation between state of health and urine pH. Wouldn't it make sense to have doctors start testing the urine pH of the patients?

8. When patients are in remission, shouldn't they be told to watch their nutrition and keep the pH balanced?

9. During chemotherapy, cancer cells as well as healthy cells are killed. As the body rebuilds itself, why not provide the ideal source of protein, with a PDCAAS score of 1?

10. Shouldn't patients be given supplements to boost their immune system?

11. I believe that a pH of 6 for urine should not be an acceptable range for a sick person as my dad was losing blood through his urine even when the pH was at 6.2. One can argue that urine pH tends to be acidic in the morning. If that is the case, shouldn't the ideal pH vary depending on what time of the day the tests were done? Logic tells me that if bleeding can occur when the urine pH is 6.2, it can never be an acceptable level for a sick patient.

We can ask many more questions. For those of you who are ready to volunteer to do the pH testing, the data you provide should be a valuable input to evidence based medicine.

Risk Factors for cancer and heart attacks.

Many people believe that certain cancers have a genetic predisposition and that there is nothing that can be done to prevent the occurrence of cancer in such people. My answer is a LOUD no. This is where the study of Nutrigenomics is essential. While you cannot change your genes, you can use proper nutrients to interact with the genes. There are DNA tests that you can take that will identify certain genes which will increase your risk to diseases. The results can provide you with personalized information and a nutrition plan to protect your health based on your DNA.

Beat Cancer Before it Beats You

If you know you have a family history of cancer and heart attack, it would be advisable to take advantage of the technological advances that are available. When you do so, I suggest you include studying Nutrigenomics.

Imagine correlating a state of good health/bad health with a reading of 24 hour pH! Following are a few studies that I can think of.

1. Charting of 24 hour pH Vs weight/BMI, body mass index.

2. Charting of 24 hour urine pH and diabetes.

3. Charting of 24 hour urine pH and cardio vascular diseases.

4. Charting of 24 hour urine pH of cancer patients through different stages of cancer therapy.

5. Charting of 24 hour urine pH of those who have recovered from cancer.

I am sure that the medical industry will come up with many based on the particular situation leading to potentially developing amazing possibilities in the treatment of diseases.

While the medical industry embrace more studies, those who are interested in improving their health can take proactive steps. The next chapter will provide a roadmap for good health and happiness.

Chapter 11

A roadmap for your good health and happiness

Now that you have read this far, I realize that you are very serious about your health. You may have many questions about the things that you have read. Here is a roadmap that I would suggest. Find your own answers to the following questions.

1. What is the baseline of your body pH? See appendix B
2. What are acid forming foods?
3. What are alkalizing foods?
4. What is acidosis and alkalosis?

Once you understand the theory behind pH balance and how your urine pH can be controlled with exercise, food habits and supplementation, you have the most useful and powerful information that can affect your health and that of everyone in your circle of influence.

Millions are affected by cancer, heart disease and much more, all degenerative diseases. Who is to be blamed? Is it the processed food industry or the pharmaceutical industry? Before we point our finger at anyone, let us look at ourselves in the mirror.

We are where we are because of all the choices that we make as human beings. God has given us the power to choose, the most powerful weapon that we have.

Beat Cancer Before it Beats You

Once you are educated on this, here is what I suggest that you do.
Follow the five step plan in maintaining the pH balance as shown in chapter 8.

.

Once your health is under control, follow the five step plan to lead a life with a purpose.

1. Write down your dreams.
2. Write down when you would like to achieve your dreams. That becomes a measurable goal.
3. Decide what you are willing to change to achieve your dreams and goals.
4. Develop a plan of action to achieve your dreams and goals.
5. Work your plan consistently and persistently.

My prayer and expectation is that God will bless you with good health and happiness and that you will share it with your loved ones.

Chapter 12

Conclusion

I would like to compare our life to a plane journey. Acidity is like the occasional turbulence that we experience in our journey. During a plane journey we are reminded to fasten our belts for our own protection. Who is there to warn us about the impending dangers to our health in this one and only journey of our life? Based on scientific evidence, pH test is our valuable tool for leading a healthy life. Just like a police force protecting the security of our communities, let the pH test be a security guard of your personal health.

I am humbled to be able to share with you something that, in my opinion, can positively affect your health for the better. Visual feedback has assisted me in watching what I consume and also for taking enough supplements as and when needed. Knowing where you are and making adjustments in the three pillars of optimal heath, lifestyle, nutrition and supplementation is what I would suggest to you as a call for action.

You may belong to one of three categories.

1. You may be an average healthy adult. Thank God every day for your health. You may ask as to why should I do pH test. The simple reason is to get a baseline and assess where you are on the pH chart. You will do it only once in your life and will convince yourself that you are on the right track occasionally. It will be rewarding to see the experimentation with different nutritional combinations and the variations

in pH. In the process you will find out what to take and what not to take.

2. You may belong to the second category, having fallen victim to some diseases. For you, it is very critical that you do your baseline following Appendix B and analyze it the way you are now. Once you know where you are, take calcium and vitamin D3, preferably from organic sources. You will be delighted to see your body getting alkalized. My expectation is that your state of health will improve. Of course, you need to consult your medical practitioner prior to taking any supplements.

3. The third category is that you may be working in the healthcare field. My hope is that the medical community will take on more research to find additional evidence correlating urine pH to many diseases. Logic tells me that the body will respond to treatments in a better way if it is neutral or alkalized than being acidic, the very principle of Homeostasis the "Milieu Interieur" espoused by Claude Bernard.

DO YOUR BEST AND GOD WILL DO THE REST.

Beat Cancer Before it Beats You

APPENDIX A

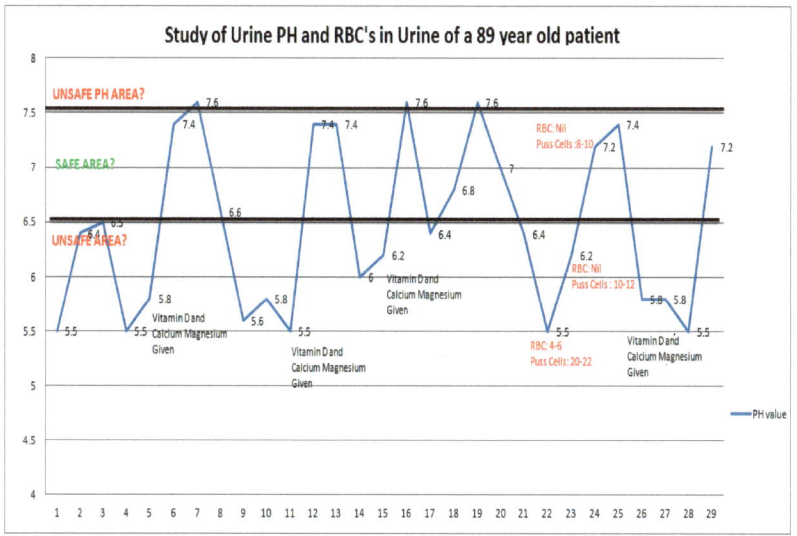

Results of tests in February 2012, immediately after diagnosis of kidney cancer. X axis give the serial number of the test and Y axis shows the urine pH measured using litmus paper.

Beat Cancer Before it Beats You

APPENDIX B

Name (Optional) _____ Age _____ Sex _____

Email (Optional)
_____

Date	Time	PH of Urine	Remarks

Urine PH ranges
4.5 to 6.0 Severely Acidotic
6.0 to 6.5 Moderately Acidotic
6.5 to 7.5 Optimal Health – Ideal pH range
7.5 and above Alkalosis

Medication if any_____

Health Condition if any_____

Please email the findings with remarks to bodyphdata@gmail.com if you would like to share the data for research purpose. Personal information is optional.

APPENDIX C

Results of Urine analysis in Jan 2013, a year after kidney cancer was detected.
Samples 7 and 8 were taken after a dose of Vitamin D3 and Calcium during lunch and also at dinner time. Acidic urine is attributed to insufficient /inadequate supplements.

#	Date	Time	Urine PH	RBC	Pus Cells	Color	Remarks
1	Jan 14, 2013	10 am	6	1-2	8-10	Normal	Blood in urine
2	Jan 14, 2013	5 pm	5.8	2-4	30-35	Normal	Blood in urine
3	Jan 15, 2013	10am	5.8	1-2	10-12	Normal	Blood in urine
4	Jan 15, 2013	5 pm	5.8	2-4	15-20	Normal	Blood in urine
5	Jan 16, 2013	11 am	6.2	1-2	10-12	Normal	Blood in urine
6	Jan17, 2013	3pm	6.2	0-1	10-12	Cloudy	Blood in urine
7	Jan18, 2013	4 am	7	0	0-1	Normal	No blood in urine
8	Jan 18, 2013	7 am	7	0	0-1	Normal	No blood in urine

Bibliography

1. *Low Urine pH: A Novel Feature of the Metabolic Syndrome.* **Naim M.Maalouf, Mary Ann Cameon, Orson W. Moe, Beverley Adams-Huet and Kashayar Sakhaee.** 2007, Clinical Journal of the American Society of Nephrology, pp. 883-888.

2. *Vitamin D3 Supplementation at 4000 Internatinal units per day for one year results in a decrease of positive cores at repeat biopsy in subjects with low-risk prostrate cancer under active surveillance.* **David T. Marshall, Stephen J. Savage, Elizabeth Garrett-Mayer, Thomas E. Keane, Bruce W. Hollis, Ronald L. Horst, Linda H. Ambrose, Mark S. Kindy, and Sebatiano Gettoni-Celli.** Charleston, SC : s.n., 2012.

3. *Dipstick measurements of Urinary pH have potential for monitoring individual and population dietary behaviors.* **Welch, A.A.** Medical school, University of East Anglia, Norwich, UK : The Open Nutrition Journal, 2008. 1874-2882/08.

4. **Anastassios G. Pittas, Tufts Medical Center.** *Vitamin D and Calcium Homeostasis for prevention of Type 2 Diabetes.* Tufts Medical Center : National Institute of Diabetes and Digestive and Kidney Diseases(NIDDK), 2011. NCT00436475.

5. **MaedaT.. Kikuchi E., Matsumoto K., Miyajima A., Oya M.** *Urinary pH is highly associated with tumor recurrence during intravesical mitomycin C therapy for nonmuscle invasive bladder tumor.* Pittsburg : National Library and the National Institutes of Health, 2011. PMID: 21239010.

6. *Urinary pH, cigarette smoking and bladder cancer risk.* **Juan Alquacil, Manolia Kogevinas, Debra T. Silverman, Nuria Malats, Francisco X. Real, Monteserrat Garcia-Closas, Adonina Tardon, Manuel Rives, Monteserrat Tora, Reina Garcia-Closas, Consol Serra, Alfredo CArrato, Ruth M.**

Pfeiffer, JOan Fortuny,..... Carcinogenesis June 2011, Bethesda, MD : Oxford Journals, 2011. 32 (6) 843-847.

7. *Influence of various beverages on urine acid output.*
Elisabeth G.E.de Vries, Coby Meyer, Marga Strubbe, et al. 430, Groningen, The Netherlands : American Association for cancer Research, 1986, Vol. 46 Jan 1986. Cancer Research 46, 430-432 January 1986.

8. **Unknown.** *Your urine is not a window to your body: pH balancing-A failed Hypothesis.* s.l. : Science based pharmacy, 2009.

9. **Wockentus AM, Koch CD, Conion PM, Sorensen LD, et al.** *Discordance between urine pH measured by dipstick and pH meter: implications for methotrexate administration protocols.* Rochester, MN, USA : Mayo Clinic, 2012. Clin biochem 2013 Jan; 46(1-2):152-4. doc 10-1016.

10. [book auth.] M.D. Michael Zimmermann. *Pocket guide to Micronutrients in Health and Disease.* Zurich : Georg Thieme Verlag, 2000.

About the Author

Thomas T. is an Electrical Engineer with a Masters degree from the Polytechnic Institute of New York. He is licensed in the state of New York as a Professional Engineer and is working as a Principal Engineer with New York City Transit Authority. He is a member of Toastmasters International having achieved the title of ACG, Advanced Communicator Gold, and is a founder of Good Souls Toastmasters in Garfield, New Jersey.

Thomas T. was born in Kerala, India and immigrated to the USA in 1980, currently living in Bloomfield, New Jersey along with Wife Maria and four children.

Beat Cancer Before it Beats You

www.ingramcontent.com/pod-product-compliance
Lightning Source LLC
Chambersburg PA
CBHW040841180526
45159CB00001B/272